1200 CALORIE DIET
TRACK YOUR DIET SUCCESS
WITH FOOD PYRAMID AND CALORIE GUIDE

Copyright 2015

Personal Goals

Start Date: _____ **End Date:** _____

My Goal:

_____

_____

_____

_____

_____

My Plan:

_____

_____

_____

_____

_____

Daily Food Target

Calories	Fat
Carbs	Fiber
Protein	Others
TOTAL	

Physical Activity Target

Daily Activity	Qty/Time
_____	_____
_____	_____
_____	_____
_____	_____

and/or

Weekly Activity	Qty/Time
_____	_____
_____	_____
_____	_____
_____	_____

My Statistics

Goal	Record one or more	Before	After	Net +/-

INFOGRAPHICS
FAST FOOD CALORIES

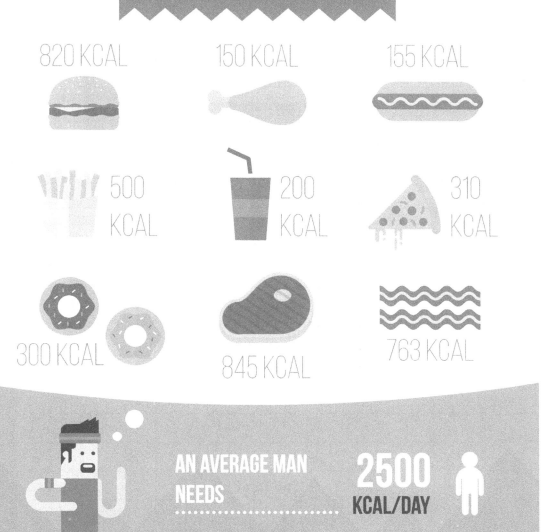

820 KCAL

150 KCAL

155 KCAL

500 KCAL

200 KCAL

310 KCAL

300 KCAL

845 KCAL

763 KCAL

AN AVERAGE MAN NEEDS .... 2500 KCAL/DAY

RUNNING BURNS ON AVERAGE .... 100 KCAL/MILE

FOOD TO AVOID?

_____

_____

_____

FOOD	QTY	CALS	CARBS	PROTEIN (g)	FAT (g)
BREAKFAST					
Sub Total					
LUNCH					
Sub Total					
DINNER					
Sub Total					
SNACK					
Sub Total					
TOTAL					

NUTRIENT	TOTAL	UNITS	GOAL %	RDA%
Calories				
Fat				
Saturated Fat				
Polyunsaturated				
Monounsaturated				

NOTES

FOOD	QTY	CALS	CARBS	PROTEIN (g)	FAT (g)
BREAKFAST					
Sub Total					
LUNCH					
Sub Total					
DINNER					
Sub Total					
SNACK					
Sub Total					
TOTAL					

NUTRIENT	TOTAL	UNITS	GOAL %	RDA%
Calories				
Fat				
Saturated Fat				
Polyunsaturated				
Monounsaturated				

NOTES

FOOD	QTY	CALS	CARBS	PROTEIN (g)	FAT (g)
BREAKFAST					
Sub Total					
LUNCH					
Sub Total					
DINNER					
Sub Total					
SNACK					
Sub Total					
TOTAL					

NUTRIENT	TOTAL	UNITS	GOAL %	RDA%
Calories				
Fat				
Saturated Fat				
Polyunsaturated				
Monounsaturated				

NOTES

FOOD	QTY	CALS	CARBS	PROTEIN (g)	FAT (g)
BREAKFAST					
Sub Total					
LUNCH					
Sub Total					
DINNER					
Sub Total					
SNACK					
Sub Total					
TOTAL					

NUTRIENT	TOTAL	UNITS	GOAL %	RDA%
Calories				
Fat				
Saturated Fat				
Polyunsaturated				
Monounsaturated				

NOTES

FOOD	QTY	CALS	CARBS	PROTEIN (g)	FAT (g)
BREAKFAST					
Sub Total					
LUNCH					
Sub Total					
DINNER					
Sub Total					
SNACK					
Sub Total					
TOTAL					

NUTRIENT	TOTAL	UNITS	GOAL %	RDA%
Calories				
Fat				
Saturated Fat				
Polyunsaturated				
Monounsaturated				

NOTES

	FOOD	QTY	CALS	CARBS	PROTEIN (g)	FAT (g)
BREAKFAST						
	Sub Total					
LUNCH						
	Sub Total					
DINNER						
	Sub Total					
SNACK						
	Sub Total					
	TOTAL					

NUTRIENT	TOTAL	UNITS	GOAL %	RDA%
Calories				
Fat				
Saturated Fat				
Polyunsaturated				
Monounsaturated				

NOTES

	FOOD	QTY	CALS	CARBS	PROTEIN (g)	FAT (g)
BREAKFAST						
	Sub Total					
LUNCH						
	Sub Total					
DINNER						
	Sub Total					
SNACK						
	Sub Total					
	TOTAL					

NUTRIENT	TOTAL	UNITS	GOAL %	RDA%
Calories				
Fat				
Saturated Fat				
Polyunsaturated				
Monounsaturated				

NOTES

	FOOD	QTY	CALS	CARBS	PROTEIN (g)	FAT (g)
BREAKFAST						
	Sub Total					
LUNCH						
	Sub Total					
DINNER						
	Sub Total					
SNACK						
	Sub Total					
	TOTAL					

NUTRIENT	TOTAL	UNITS	GOAL %	RDA%
Calories				
Fat				
Saturated Fat				
Polyunsaturated				
Monounsaturated				

NOTES

FOOD	QTY	CALS	CARBS	PROTEIN (g)	FAT (g)
BREAKFAST					
Sub Total					
LUNCH					
Sub Total					
DINNER					
Sub Total					
SNACK					
Sub Total					
TOTAL					

NUTRIENT	TOTAL	UNITS	GOAL %	RDA%
Calories				
Fat				
Saturated Fat				
Polyunsaturated				
Monounsaturated				

NOTES

	FOOD	QTY	CALS	CARBS	PROTEIN (g)	FAT (g)
BREAKFAST						
	Sub Total					
LUNCH						
	Sub Total					
DINNER						
	Sub Total					
SNACK						
	Sub Total					
	TOTAL					

NUTRIENT	TOTAL	UNITS	GOAL %	RDA%
Calories				
Fat				
Saturated Fat				
Polyunsaturated				
Monounsaturated				

NOTES

FOOD	QTY	CALS	CARBS	PROTEIN (g)	FAT (g)
BREAKFAST					
Sub Total					
LUNCH					
Sub Total					
DINNER					
Sub Total					
SNACK					
Sub Total					
TOTAL					

NUTRIENT	TOTAL	UNITS	GOAL %	RDA%
Calories				
Fat				
Saturated Fat				
Polyunsaturated				
Monounsaturated				

NOTES

FOOD	QTY	CALS	CARBS	PROTEIN (g)	FAT (g)
BREAKFAST					
Sub Total					
LUNCH					
Sub Total					
DINNER					
Sub Total					
SNACK					
Sub Total					
TOTAL					

NUTRIENT	TOTAL	UNITS	GOAL %	RDA%
Calories				
Fat				
Saturated Fat				
Polyunsaturated				
Monounsaturated				

GRAINS

VEGETABLES

FRUITS

FAT

MILK

MEAT & BEANS

FOOD	QTY	CALS	CARBS	PROTEIN (g)	FAT (g)
BREAKFAST					
Sub Total					
LUNCH					
Sub Total					
DINNER					
Sub Total					
SNACK					
Sub Total					
TOTAL					

NUTRIENT	TOTAL	UNITS	GOAL %	RDA%
Calories				
Fat				
Saturated Fat				
Polyunsaturated				
Monounsaturated				

NOTES

	FOOD	QTY	CALS	CARBS	PROTEIN (g)	FAT (g)
BREAKFAST						
	Sub Total					
LUNCH						
	Sub Total					
DINNER						
	Sub Total					
SNACK						
	Sub Total					
	TOTAL					

NUTRIENT	TOTAL	UNITS	GOAL %	RDA%
Calories				
Fat				
Saturated Fat				
Polyunsaturated				
Monounsaturated				

NOTES

	FOOD	QTY	CALS	CARBS	PROTEIN (g)	FAT (g)
BREAKFAST						
	Sub Total					
LUNCH						
	Sub Total					
DINNER						
	Sub Total					
SNACK						
	Sub Total					
	TOTAL					

NUTRIENT	TOTAL	UNITS	GOAL %	RDA%
Calories				
Fat				
Saturated Fat				
Polyunsaturated				
Monounsaturated				

NOTES

	FOOD	QTY	CALS	CARBS	PROTEIN (g)	FAT (g)
BREAKFAST						
	Sub Total					
LUNCH						
	Sub Total					
DINNER						
	Sub Total					
SNACK						
	Sub Total					
	TOTAL					

NUTRIENT	TOTAL	UNITS	GOAL %	RDA%
Calories				
Fat				
Saturated Fat				
Polyunsaturated				
Monounsaturated				

NOTES

	FOOD	QTY	CALS	CARBS	PROTEIN (g)	FAT (g)
BREAKFAST						
	Sub Total					
LUNCH						
	Sub Total					
DINNER						
	Sub Total					
SNACK						
	Sub Total					
	TOTAL					

NUTRIENT	TOTAL	UNITS	GOAL %	RDA%
Calories				
Fat				
Saturated Fat				
Polyunsaturated				
Monounsaturated				

NOTES

FOOD	QTY	CALS	CARBS	PROTEIN (g)	FAT (g)
BREAKFAST					
Sub Total					
LUNCH					
Sub Total					
DINNER					
Sub Total					
SNACK					
Sub Total					
TOTAL					

NUTRIENT	TOTAL	UNITS	GOAL %	RDA%
Calories				
Fat				
Saturated Fat				
Polyunsaturated				
Monounsaturated				

NOTES

FOOD	QTY	CALS	CARBS	PROTEIN (g)	FAT (g)
BREAKFAST					
Sub Total					
LUNCH					
Sub Total					
DINNER					
Sub Total					
SNACK					
Sub Total					
TOTAL					

NUTRIENT	TOTAL	UNITS	GOAL %	RDA%
Calories				
Fat				
Saturated Fat				
Polyunsaturated				
Monounsaturated				

NOTES

	FOOD	QTY	CALS	CARBS	PROTEIN (g)	FAT (g)
BREAKFAST						
	Sub Total					
LUNCH						
	Sub Total					
DINNER						
	Sub Total					
SNACK						
	Sub Total					
	TOTAL					

NUTRIENT	TOTAL	UNITS	GOAL %	RDA%
Calories				
Fat				
Saturated Fat				
Polyunsaturated				
Monounsaturated				

NOTES

	FOOD	QTY	CALS	CARBS	PROTEIN (g)	FAT (g)
BREAKFAST						
	Sub Total					
LUNCH						
	Sub Total					
DINNER						
	Sub Total					
SNACK						
	Sub Total					
	TOTAL					

NUTRIENT	TOTAL	UNITS	GOAL %	RDA%
Calories				
Fat				
Saturated Fat				
Polyunsaturated				
Monounsaturated				

NOTES

FOOD	QTY	CALS	CARBS	PROTEIN (g)	FAT (g)
BREAKFAST					
Sub Total					
LUNCH					
Sub Total					
DINNER					
Sub Total					
SNACK					
Sub Total					
TOTAL					

NUTRIENT	TOTAL	UNITS	GOAL %	RDA%
Calories				
Fat				
Saturated Fat				
Polyunsaturated				
Monounsaturated				

NOTES

FOOD	QTY	CALS	CARBS	PROTEIN (g)	FAT (g)
BREAKFAST					
Sub Total					
LUNCH					
Sub Total					
DINNER					
Sub Total					
SNACK					
Sub Total					
TOTAL					

NUTRIENT	TOTAL	UNITS	GOAL %	RDA%
Calories				
Fat				
Saturated Fat				
Polyunsaturated				
Monounsaturated				

NOTES

	FOOD	QTY	CALS	CARBS	PROTEIN (g)	FAT (g)
BREAKFAST						
	Sub Total					
LUNCH						
	Sub Total					
DINNER						
	Sub Total					
SNACK						
	Sub Total					
	TOTAL					

NUTRIENT	TOTAL	UNITS	GOAL %	RDA%
Calories				
Fat				
Saturated Fat				
Polyunsaturated				
Monounsaturated				

NOTES

	FOOD	QTY	CALS	CARBS	PROTEIN (g)	FAT (g)
BREAKFAST						
	Sub Total					
LUNCH						
	Sub Total					
DINNER						
	Sub Total					
SNACK						
	Sub Total					
	TOTAL					

NUTRIENT	TOTAL	UNITS	GOAL %	RDA%
Calories				
Fat				
Saturated Fat				
Polyunsaturated				
Monounsaturated				

NOTES

	FOOD	QTY	CALS	CARBS	PROTEIN (g)	FAT (g)
BREAKFAST						
	Sub Total					
LUNCH						
	Sub Total					
DINNER						
	Sub Total					
SNACK						
	Sub Total					
	TOTAL					

NUTRIENT	TOTAL	UNITS	GOAL %	RDA%
Calories				
Fat				
Saturated Fat				
Polyunsaturated				
Monounsaturated				

NOTES

FOOD	QTY	CALS	CARBS	PROTEIN (g)	FAT (g)
BREAKFAST					
Sub Total					
LUNCH					
Sub Total					
DINNER					
Sub Total					
SNACK					
Sub Total					
TOTAL					

NUTRIENT	TOTAL	UNITS	GOAL %	RDA%
Calories				
Fat				
Saturated Fat				
Polyunsaturated				
Monounsaturated				

NOTES

	FOOD	QTY	CALS	CARBS	PROTEIN (g)	FAT (g)
BREAKFAST						
	Sub Total					
LUNCH						
	Sub Total					
DINNER						
	Sub Total					
SNACK						
	Sub Total					
	TOTAL					

NUTRIENT	TOTAL	UNITS	GOAL %	RDA%
Calories				
Fat				
Saturated Fat				
Polyunsaturated				
Monounsaturated				

NOTES

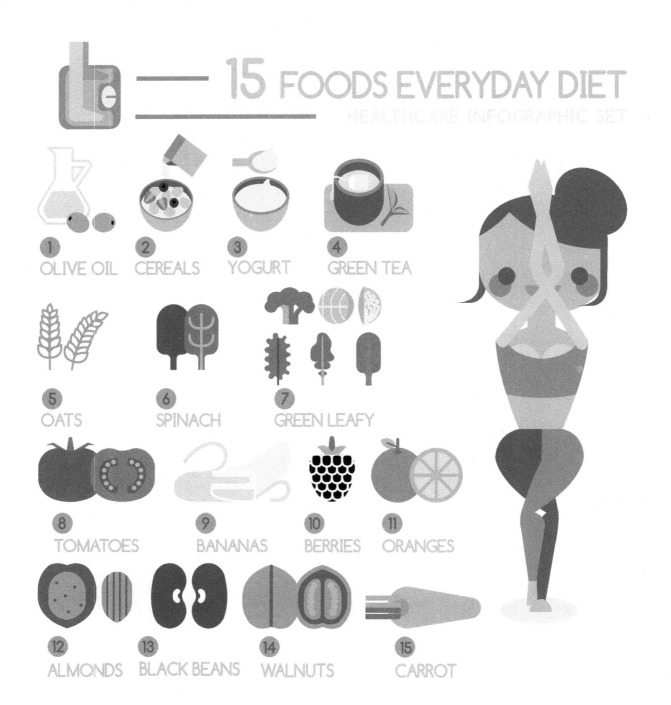

15 FOODS EVERYDAY DIET

HEALTHCARE INFOGRAPHIC SET

1 OLIVE OIL
2 CEREALS
3 YOGURT
4 GREEN TEA
5 OATS
6 SPINACH
7 GREEN LEAFY
8 TOMATOES
9 BANANAS
10 BERRIES
11 ORANGES
12 ALMONDS
13 BLACK BEANS
14 WALNUTS
15 CARROT

THINGS TO REMEMBER:

_____

_____

_____

_____

_____

NOTES

	FOOD	QTY	CALS	CARBS	PROTEIN (g)	FAT (g)
BREAKFAST						
	Sub Total					
LUNCH						
	Sub Total					
DINNER						
	Sub Total					
SNACK						
	Sub Total					
	TOTAL					

NUTRIENT	TOTAL	UNITS	GOAL %	RDA%
Calories				
Fat				
Saturated Fat				
Polyunsaturated				
Monounsaturated				

NOTES

	FOOD	QTY	CALS	CARBS	PROTEIN (g)	FAT (g)
BREAKFAST						
	Sub Total					
LUNCH						
	Sub Total					
DINNER						
	Sub Total					
SNACK						
	Sub Total					
	TOTAL					

NUTRIENT	TOTAL	UNITS	GOAL %	RDA%
Calories				
Fat				
Saturated Fat				
Polyunsaturated				
Monounsaturated				

NOTES

	FOOD	QTY	CALS	CARBS	PROTEIN (g)	FAT (g)
BREAKFAST						
	Sub Total					
LUNCH						
	Sub Total					
DINNER						
	Sub Total					
SNACK						
	Sub Total					
	TOTAL					

NUTRIENT	TOTAL	UNITS	GOAL %	RDA%
Calories				
Fat				
Saturated Fat				
Polyunsaturated				
Monounsaturated				

NOTES

FOOD	QTY	CALS	CARBS	PROTEIN (g)	FAT (g)
BREAKFAST					
Sub Total					
LUNCH					
Sub Total					
DINNER					
Sub Total					
SNACK					
Sub Total					
TOTAL					

NUTRIENT	TOTAL	UNITS	GOAL %	RDA%
Calories				
Fat				
Saturated Fat				
Polyunsaturated				
Monounsaturated				

NOTES

	FOOD	QTY	CALS	CARBS	PROTEIN (g)	FAT (g)
BREAKFAST						
	Sub Total					
LUNCH						
	Sub Total					
DINNER						
	Sub Total					
SNACK						
	Sub Total					
	TOTAL					

NUTRIENT	TOTAL	UNITS	GOAL %	RDA%
Calories				
Fat				
Saturated Fat				
Polyunsaturated				
Monounsaturated				

NOTES

	FOOD	QTY	CALS	CARBS	PROTEIN (g)	FAT (g)
BREAKFAST						
	Sub Total					
LUNCH						
	Sub Total					
DINNER						
	Sub Total					
SNACK						
	Sub Total					
	TOTAL					

NUTRIENT	TOTAL	UNITS	GOAL %	RDA%
Calories				
Fat				
Saturated Fat				
Polyunsaturated				
Monounsaturated				

NOTES

	FOOD	QTY	CALS	CARBS	PROTEIN (g)	FAT (g)
BREAKFAST						
	Sub Total					
LUNCH						
	Sub Total					
DINNER						
	Sub Total					
SNACK						
	Sub Total					
	TOTAL					

NUTRIENT	TOTAL	UNITS	GOAL %	RDA%
Calories				
Fat				
Saturated Fat				
Polyunsaturated				
Monounsaturated				

NOTES

	FOOD	QTY	CALS	CARBS	PROTEIN (g)	FAT (g)
BREAKFAST						
	Sub Total					
LUNCH						
	Sub Total					
DINNER						
	Sub Total					
SNACK						
	Sub Total					
	TOTAL					

NUTRIENT	TOTAL	UNITS	GOAL %	RDA%
Calories				
Fat				
Saturated Fat				
Polyunsaturated				
Monounsaturated				

NOTES

FOOD	QTY	CALS	CARBS	PROTEIN (g)	FAT (g)
BREAKFAST					
Sub Total					
LUNCH					
Sub Total					
DINNER					
Sub Total					
SNACK					
Sub Total					
TOTAL					

NUTRIENT	TOTAL	UNITS	GOAL %	RDA%
Calories				
Fat				
Saturated Fat				
Polyunsaturated				
Monounsaturated				

NOTES

4 SIMPLE STEP TO WELLNESS

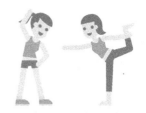

HEALTHY DIET	REGULAR EXERCISE	RELAXATION	PLENTY OF REST

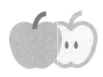

NUTRITIOUS FOOD

IMPROVES ALERTNESS AND CREATIVITY

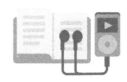

MUSIC OR READ THE BOOK BEFORE BED TO HELP PROMOTE RESTFUL SLEEP

PROPER SLEEP WILL HELP YOU STAY ATTENTIVE AND ACTIVE

DON'T SKIP BREAKFAST

IMPROVES YOUR PHYSICAL AND MENTAL WELL-BEING

AVOID USING ALCOHOL TO RELAX ESPECIALLY BEFORE BED

A LACK OF SLEEP WILL CAUSE YOU TO HAVE TO WORK HARDER TO GET DAILY TASKS DONE

AVOID EXCESSIVE AMOUNTS OF CAFFEINE

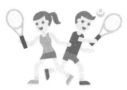

KEEPS YOU ACTIVE AND SOCIAL

LAUGHING DECREASES PAIN, PROMOTES MUSCLE RELAXATION AND CAN REDUCE ANXIETY

A CONTINUED LACK OF SLEEP CAN LEAD TO MOOD CHANGES, ANXIETY, AND LOWERED RESISTANCE TO ILLNESS

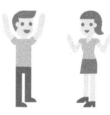

KEEP YOUR BODY ENERGIZED

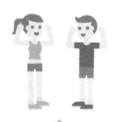

ELEVATES YOUR MOOD, REDUCES STRESS, INCREASE ENERGY, AND RAISES YOUR ENDORPHIN LEVELS

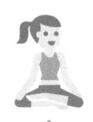

QUALITY RELAXATION HELP YOU DISCONNECT FROM YOUR PROBLEMS AND OFFERS A SENSE OF COMPETENCE

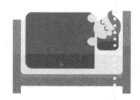

ADEQUATE SLEEP ALLOWS YOU TO COPE WITH THE PSYCHOLOGICAL AND PHYSICAL AND PHYSICAL STRESSORS OF DAILY LIFE

MY GOAL:

_____

_____

_____

_____

_____

NOTES

	FOOD	QTY	CALS	CARBS	PROTEIN (g)	FAT (g)
BREAKFAST						
	Sub Total					
LUNCH						
	Sub Total					
DINNER						
	Sub Total					
SNACK						
	Sub Total					
	TOTAL					

NUTRIENT	TOTAL	UNITS	GOAL %	RDA%
Calories				
Fat				
Saturated Fat				
Polyunsaturated				
Monounsaturated				

NOTES

FOOD	QTY	CALS	CARBS	PROTEIN (g)	FAT (g)
BREAKFAST					
Sub Total					
LUNCH					
Sub Total					
DINNER					
Sub Total					
SNACK					
Sub Total					
TOTAL					

NUTRIENT	TOTAL	UNITS	GOAL %	RDA%
Calories				
Fat				
Saturated Fat				
Polyunsaturated				
Monounsaturated				

NOTES

	FOOD	QTY	CALS	CARBS	PROTEIN (g)	FAT (g)
BREAKFAST						
	Sub Total					
LUNCH						
	Sub Total					
DINNER						
	Sub Total					
SNACK						
	Sub Total					
	TOTAL					

NUTRIENT	TOTAL	UNITS	GOAL %	RDA%
Calories				
Fat				
Saturated Fat				
Polyunsaturated				
Monounsaturated				

NOTES

	FOOD	QTY	CALS	CARBS	PROTEIN (g)	FAT (g)
BREAKFAST						
	Sub Total					
LUNCH						
	Sub Total					
DINNER						
	Sub Total					
SNACK						
	Sub Total					
	TOTAL					

NUTRIENT	TOTAL	UNITS	GOAL %	RDA%
Calories				
Fat				
Saturated Fat				
Polyunsaturated				
Monounsaturated				

NOTES

FOOD	QTY	CALS	CARBS	PROTEIN (g)	FAT (g)
BREAKFAST					
Sub Total					
LUNCH					
Sub Total					
DINNER					
Sub Total					
SNACK					
Sub Total					
TOTAL					

NUTRIENT	TOTAL	UNITS	GOAL %	RDA%
Calories				
Fat				
Saturated Fat				
Polyunsaturated				
Monounsaturated				

NOTES

	FOOD	QTY	CALS	CARBS	PROTEIN (g)	FAT (g)
BREAKFAST						
	Sub Total					
LUNCH						
	Sub Total					
DINNER						
	Sub Total					
SNACK						
	Sub Total					
	TOTAL					

NUTRIENT	TOTAL	UNITS	GOAL %	RDA%
Calories				
Fat				
Saturated Fat				
Polyunsaturated				
Monounsaturated				

NOTES

	FOOD	QTY	CALS	CARBS	PROTEIN (g)	FAT (g)
BREAKFAST						
	Sub Total					
LUNCH						
	Sub Total					
DINNER						
	Sub Total					
SNACK						
	Sub Total					
	TOTAL					

NUTRIENT	TOTAL	UNITS	GOAL %	RDA%
Calories				
Fat				
Saturated Fat				
Polyunsaturated				
Monounsaturated				

NOTES

	FOOD	QTY	CALS	CARBS	PROTEIN (g)	FAT (g)
BREAKFAST						
	Sub Total					
LUNCH						
	Sub Total					
DINNER						
	Sub Total					
SNACK						
	Sub Total					
	TOTAL					

NUTRIENT	TOTAL	UNITS	GOAL %	RDA%
Calories				
Fat				
Saturated Fat				
Polyunsaturated				
Monounsaturated				

NOTES

	FOOD	QTY	CALS	CARBS	PROTEIN (g)	FAT (g)
BREAKFAST						
	Sub Total					
LUNCH						
	Sub Total					
DINNER						
	Sub Total					
SNACK						
	Sub Total					
	TOTAL					

NUTRIENT	TOTAL	UNITS	GOAL %	RDA%
Calories				
Fat				
Saturated Fat				
Polyunsaturated				
Monounsaturated				

NOTES

	FOOD	QTY	CALS	CARBS	PROTEIN (g)	FAT (g)
BREAKFAST						
	Sub Total					
LUNCH						
	Sub Total					
DINNER						
	Sub Total					
SNACK						
	Sub Total					
	TOTAL					

NUTRIENT	TOTAL	UNITS	GOAL %	RDA%
Calories				
Fat				
Saturated Fat				
Polyunsaturated				
Monounsaturated				

NOTES

	FOOD	QTY	CALS	CARBS	PROTEIN (g)	FAT (g)
BREAKFAST						
	Sub Total					
LUNCH						
	Sub Total					
DINNER						
	Sub Total					
SNACK						
	Sub Total					
	TOTAL					

NUTRIENT	TOTAL	UNITS	GOAL %	RDA%
Calories				
Fat				
Saturated Fat				
Polyunsaturated				
Monounsaturated				

NOTES

CPSIA information can be obtained
at www.ICGtesting.com
Printed in the USA
LVHW061935250723
753095LV00011B/294